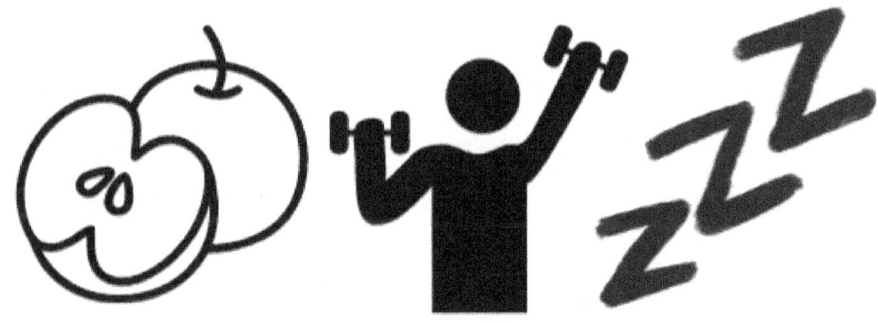

LAZY BUT HEALTHY

Health & Legal Disclaimer

The information provided in this book, including advice and recipes, is intended for general informational purposes only and is not a substitute for professional medical advice, diagnosis, or treatment. Always seek the advice of your physician or other qualified health provider with any questions you may have regarding a medical condition.

The author of this book is not a medical professional, and the content presented here is based on personal experimentation and research. While every effort has been made to ensure the accuracy and completeness of the information provided, the author makes no representations or warranties of any kind, express or implied, about the suitability or effectiveness of the information for any specific purpose.

The author disclaims any liability or responsibility for any loss or damage that may arise from reliance on the information contained in this book. It is essential to consult with a healthcare professional before making any significant changes to your diet, exercise routine, or health-related practices, especially if you have underlying medical conditions or are taking medication.

Any health-related recommendations, tips, or recipes provided in this book should be considered as suggestions and not as medical advice. Readers are encouraged to use their discretion and consult with healthcare professionals to make informed decisions about their health and well-being.

By reading and using the information in this book, you acknowledge and agree to these terms and conditions. Your health is a personal matter, and it is essential to take responsibility for it by consulting with qualified healthcare professionals as needed. Always prioritize your health and safety above all else.

Copyright © [2023] by [Miguel Recommends]

All rights reserved. No part of this book may be reproduced, distributed, or transmitted in any form or by any means, including photocopying, recording, or other electronic or mechanical methods, without the prior written permission of the publisher, except in the case of brief quotations embodied in critical reviews and certain other noncommercial uses permitted by copyright law.

For permission requests, write to the publisher at: Amazon

This book is a work of non-fiction. Names, characters, places, and incidents either are the product of the author's imagination or are used fictitiously. Any resemblance to actual persons, living or dead, events, or locales is entirely coincidental.

I dedicate this book to:

Obviously, you, that bought this book. My goal in life is to work smarter, not harder and this is the main theme of this cookbook. The fact that you purchased the book is a sign and testament that you want to do things right, but at the same time are kind of not in the full mood to do so. Thank you.

Table of Contents

Prologue 6

Introduction 7

About Me 8

Breakfasts 11

Anabolic French Toast 12

French Toast Egg Sando 14

PROATMEAL Breakfast 15

Omelet (Tex-Mex Style) 17

Protein Pancake 18

(Banana Style) 18

Omelet (Ham & Cheese) 20

Egg White Avo Toast & 21

Egg Avo Toast 21

Egg White Bites 23

Protein Muffins (Blueberry) 24

Lunch 26

Chili Chicken Rice Bowls: 27

QUESADILLA 29

TACO PASTA 31

Chipotle Chicken & Rice 33

Vegan Meatball Sub 35

Deconstructed Cheeseburger 36

Open Face Chicken Sando x2 38

Snacks & Appetizers 39

Popcorn 40

PeaNOT Butter cupcakes 41

RICE CAKES! 42

Protein Fruit Ice Cream 43

Cauliflower mash 44

Egg white fries 46

Homemade Chicken Nuggets 48

DINNERS 50

Swed(ish) Meatballs 51

Citrusy Tilapia and Shrimp 53

Baked salmon & Long Greens 54

PIZZA A LA PROTEINA 56

Epilogue 57

Prologue

Thank you for your time! I hope all the knowledge I have collected throughout the years regarding weight loss and food and stuff helps you. I'm no doctor, but I think I kinda figured it out.

One thing I do want to address right off the bat. It is not easy. There are no shortcuts. You need to have the will to improve, and it takes a while to change that mindset and break from habits that you have already gotten used to.

Diets fail. Let's be honest about this. Who hasn't started 'keto', 'Atkins', this and the other to then going back to the old ways? I know I have, for years on end. You'll notice in this book I won't add much 'before' pictures of me, if any. The reason for this is that I am 5'8'' and got as heavy as 205 lbs., which is, in my opinion, a bit overweight to say the least. I started measuring what I ate, moving around more and think I can explain in more detail all of this.

What inspired me to write this book? Well, first and foremost, I have always been lazy and consider myself pretty good as explaining things. The fact that I can transmit this information and knowledge I have tried myself to improve even if it just one more person, it is all worth it. All of this because I want people to feel as good as I have felt ever since I have been in a normal more manageable weight!

Sadly, we live in a society that is good at misleading and selling stuff that won't work. My goal is to present to you my thoughts that have worked for me and friends and family I have suggested the things I will go over this cookbook.

It's a cookbook you will have handy for some time as I believe I will provide really good information that will help you for years ahead.

Introduction

First things first. Your brain should be already shifted and focused on one thing: Losing weight. If your brain is already in sync with this, we can go ahead and start.

The main point on this book is to rewire how you see nutrition and overall health. I'll try to explain in simple and sometimes (hopefully) funny ways to approach things in life. The core principles that I will go over are just 3 plain and simple ones. Watch what you eat, move around and sleep well. Think of us as sharks, if they stop moving/swimming, they'll die.

I get it, I am lazy, but not that dumb, so I decided to sit down and think of a way to figure it out. I think I did. The main goal is to show you a couple of recipes that have helped me to lose weight.

How did I do it? Well, I sat down one day and counted what I ate and how much I moved. I ate a lot and didn't move much (of course, being lazy), so I changed it. I started replacing one meal of the day to one of these listed in this cookbook, then 2 and then 3.

I get it, you don't do 3, you do 5, you do keto, you do Atkins, you are lactose intolerant, you do fasting and so on. I have tried to put enough recipes here to match all those boxes. You will find keto, you also can change ingredients, but make sure to count the calories, as it is the base for everything. You want to try to eat as many grams of protein as your body weight. Why protein? It is the one that the body has the most fun digesting and takes it time to do so. It will basically keep you fuller for longer.

Another goal is to try to make food taste as good as the real thing, but by using healthier or low-calorie dense food. I will provide what I think is the difficulty level from 1 star to 3 stars and explain if one is for bulk cooking and all the dietary details at the end.

Lastly, please realize I am not a doctor and even if you start losing weight by changing your diet, there will be a moment where you will plateau. What do you do then? Move more. Start being more active. This will make you hungrier and you will eat more from this cookbook.

About Me

So, you've already read some pages about me yapping about moving and calories and how fat I was and how good I have this thing going on now, but at the end of the day, who am I?

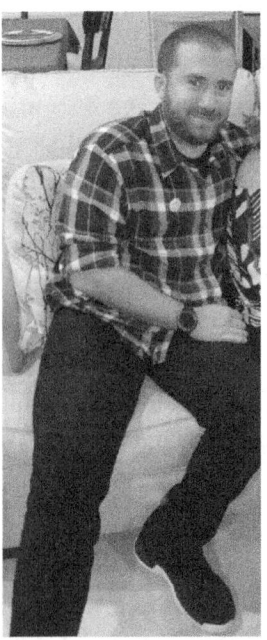
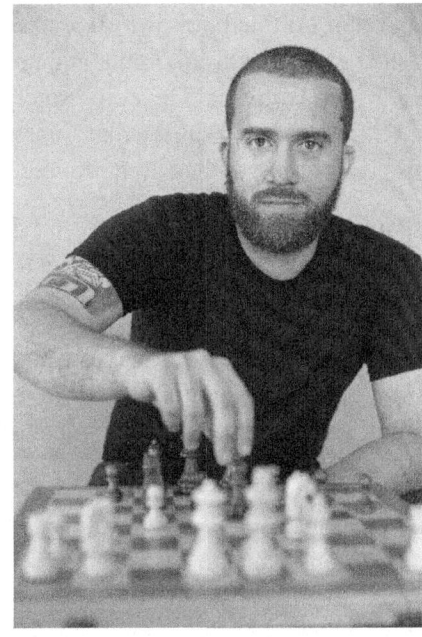

I have always found it difficult to talk about me, but here we go I suppose. My name is Miguel Lora, and I was originally born in the Dominican Republic, been living in the USA for over 10 years. I reside in the best state ever, Florida, and my family does live here as well.

I am an Electrical Engineer according to my degree, but I am just a fan of trying to make sense out of things. I enjoy watching movies, listening to music, and reading all sorts of things from philosophy to basically strip comics. Make sure to check my sites if you want to know what I talk about there:

SITE: www.Miguelrecs.com

As mentioned, I was born in the Caribbean, grew up over there and my first language is Spanish. I will probably publish a Spanish version of this book soon.

I share my house with these 2 fellas: Leo & Layla, my cats!

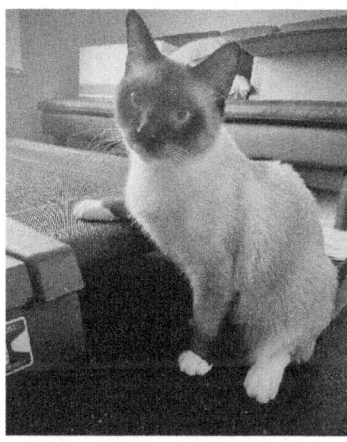 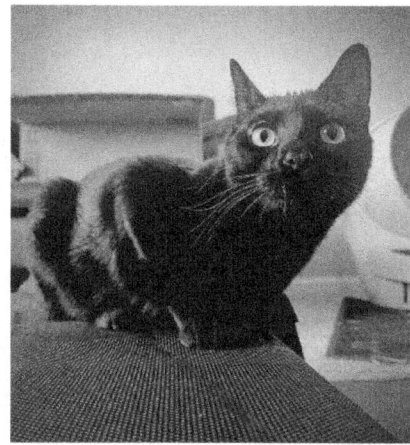

They were the ones that convinced me to write this book and publish it as they have been witnesses to my weight loss journey and look at me like I am insane as you can see.

You can also see on those pictures that I was getting a bit heavy. I realized this when I went for my annual doctor visit and the doctor told me to open my mouth and say 'oink'. That was my wake-up call.

I was a Field Engineer an all that traveling made me eat out all the time and completely disregard my health, habits were eating crappy food. This cookbook is my representation of my efforts and to show you stuff that works.

Breakfasts

Anabolic French Toast

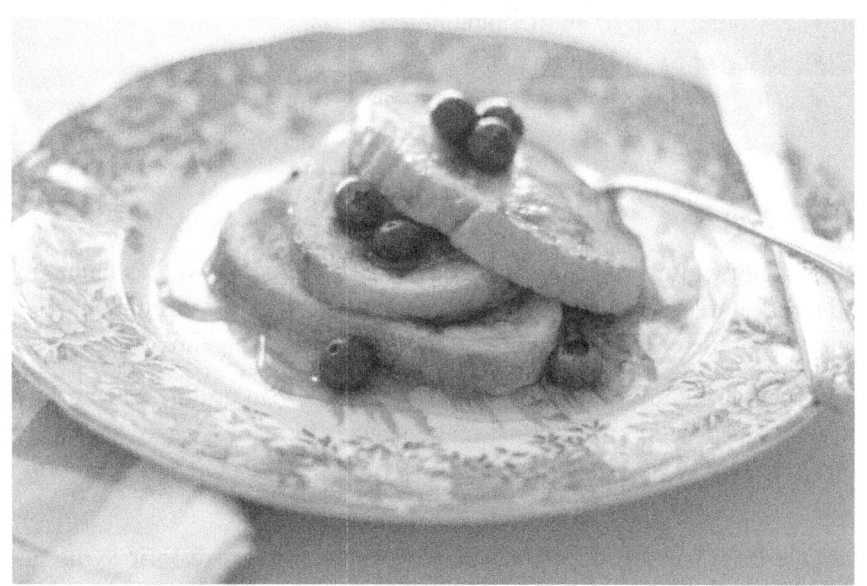

This is one of my favorite recipes to make. Why? It's easy, nutritious, and will keep you full for a while, and in contrast, being low on calories. I will provide all the details at the end. Check this one out:

Difficulty: ✪

Ingredients

- 3/4 cup or 180g of egg whites
- 2 slices of white bread (around 70/80 calories per slice of bread)
- 2 packets of sweetener (I use stevia)
- Around 1 tsp or 3g of Cinnamon
- 1 tsp or 5g of Vanilla extract
- 4tbsp or 60 ml of low-calorie maple syrup.

Preparation

Mix the egg whites, sweetener packets, vanilla extract as well as cinnamon and whisk until everything is incorporated and distributed throughout. Heat a pan or griddle over medium to low heat and spray with cooking spray.

Dip bread slices into the mixture and transfer to pan/griddle. If you have leftover egg mixture, throw it over the slices of bread that are cooking. If you do it slowly, the bread should absorb all of it. Cook 3 to 4 mins per side.

Remove from pan and serve on a plate, top with the low-calorie syrup and fresh fruit. I like Strawberries and blueberries with mine. That's it.

This amazing dish is 270 calories, 1g of fat, 30g of carbs, 6g of fiber, and 28g of protein! This will keep you full for longer while being low on calories and high on protein.

French Toast Egg Sando

This one will make you full. Trust me.

Difficulty: ✪✪

Ingredients

- 2 slices of bread
- 2 slices of fat free cheese
- 2 cups or 480g of egg whites
- Salt and pepper for seasoning, maybe no sugar ketchup as a condiment

Preparation

Heat nonstick pan on medium heat, spray with cooking spray and pour egg white mixture (seasoned with salt and pepper)

Place bread slices for 15 to 20 seconds, then flip (this will make the bread drench in the egg white mixture) continue to cook and then flip, proceed to fold the egg onto bread while placing the slices of cheese inside.

The macros for this dish should be approximately like this: 480 cal 3g of fat, 40g carbs, 2g fiber & 69g protein.

__PROATMEAL Breakfast__

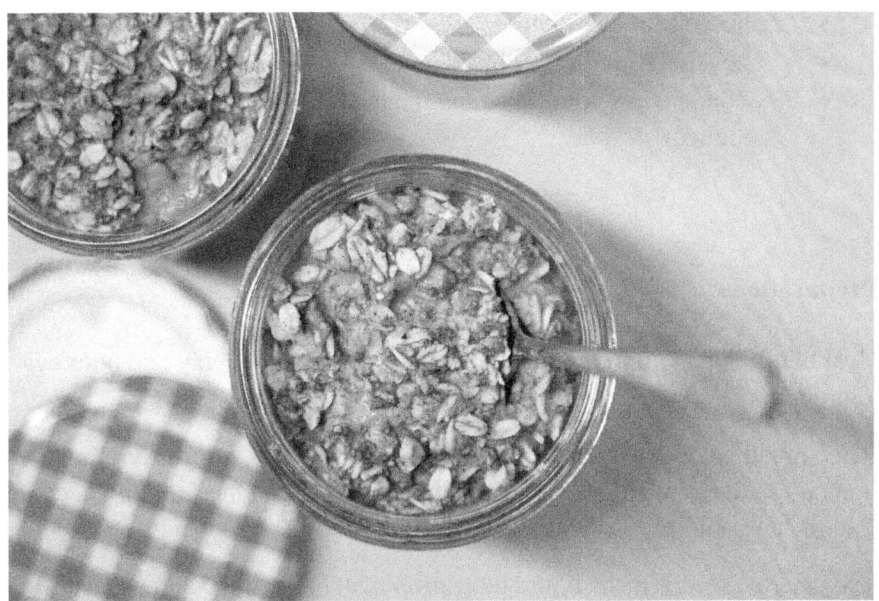

Difficulty: zero stars.

This is a recipe that I have used on my lazier days either for breakfast or dinner. It has helped me during my weight loss journey, and is incredibly rich, as it will provide you with Protein, meaning that it will keep you full for longer while being low on calories and high on Protein.

Ingredients:

- Old Fashioned Oatmeal (1/2 cup -approx. 150 calories)
- Chia Seeds (1 Tbsp -approx. 70 calories)
- Water (1 cup – 0 calories)
- Protein Powder (1 scoop -approx. 110 calories)
- Cinnamon powder (for extra taste)

Preparation:

Easiest preparation ever. Pour 1/cup of the Old-Fashioned oatmeal grains into a cup or a vessel where you're going to be eating this amazing dish. Then add one cup of water, then a scoop of protein powder, and then a Tbsp of Chia seeds.

Proceed to mix all the ingredients thoroughly until everything is well incorporated.

Then put it in the fridge for around 10 mins and the chia seeds will make the mixture denser and thicker, kind of like ice cream, then you can add some Cinnamon powder for extra sweetness and that's it!

You'll get a nice hearty ice cream-like meal for around 300 calories that will keep you full and provide you with very-needed fiber and protein.

Omelet (Tex-Mex Style)

This one is gluten free and ready in 15 mins or so.

Difficulty: ✪✪

Ingredients:

- 150g or 3/4 cup of egg whites.
- 1 egg
- 2 slices of cheese (fat free)
- 110g or 4oz of lean ground beef (you can use turkey if you want, but make sure its lean)
- 110g of tomato diced.
- 60g yellow onion diced.
- 60g red bell pepper diced.
- 10g green onion diced.
- Salt, pepper, chili powder and ground cumin to taste.

Preparation

In a nonstick pan, cook the ground meat, then drain excess fat, remove from pan. Sautee all vegetables in pan until desired consistency and add the cooked ground meat prepared before.

Separately in a bowl, whisk egg whites and egg and add all other ingredients and mix well and then add to meat and vegetables. Continue to cook for 3 mins or until egg white mixture, you know the drill to make omelet, until everything is settled then flip to the other side and repeat.

Once fully cooked, just serve and add some toppings like salsa or sour cream (fat free)!

This will add to around 400 calories or so, 8g of fat, 28g of carps, 5g of fiber and 50g of protein or so.

Protein Pancake (Banana Style)

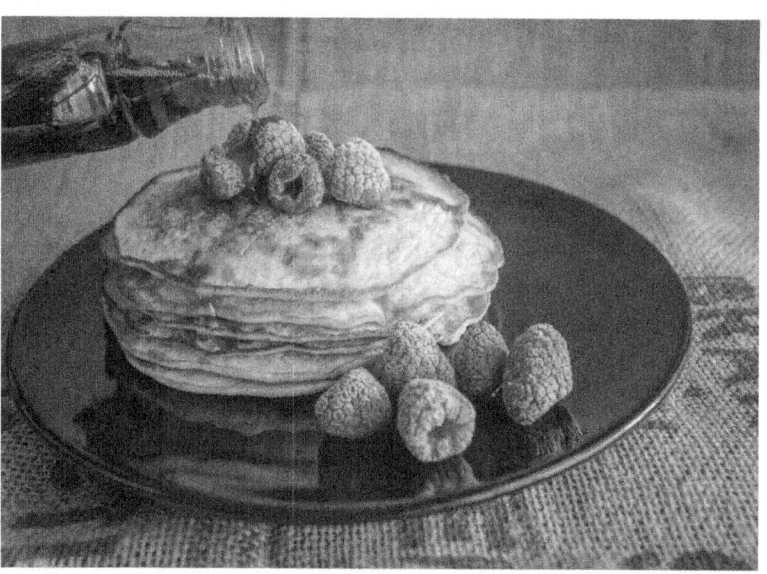

This Vegetarian and Gluten free recipe is easy and read in like 10 to 15 minutes.

Difficulty: ✪

Ingredients

- 180g or 3/4 cup of egg whites.
- 200g of banana
- 1 scoop of protein powder of preference
- 65g or 3/4 cup of rolled oats.
- 15g cocoa powder
- 1 tsp cinnamon
- Top w/ 4tbsp of low-cal syrup

Preparation

Add all ingredients to a power blender and blend until the consistency is the same all around (around a minute or so) and transfer to let thicken for a little bit.

Heat a skillet over medium to high heat, spray with cooking spray and add batter. Cook each side for 3 or 4 mins, then flip. Do this for all 4 servings and if you want, you can save the batter for later.

This batch will have around 700 calories, 8g of fat, 100 carbs, 15g of fiber and 58 of protein.

Each pancake should be around 180 calories, 2g of fat, 27g of carbs, 4g of fiber and approx. 15g of protein.

Omelet (Ham & Cheese)

This one is relatively easy, gluten free and ready in 10 mins.

Difficulty: ✪

Ingredients

- 480g or 2 ups of egg whites
- 100 lean deli ham diced.
- mixed veggies, spinach, tomatoes, onions
- 4 slices or 70g of shredded fat free cheese
- salt and pepper

Preparation:

Whisk egg whites in a bowl and add all mixed veggies and mix well

Using a nonstick pan on medium heat, spray with cooking spray and add mixture to cook one side for 3 minutes or so (until partially cooked) then add 2 slices of the cheese, fold over and cook for 2 or 3 more mins while adding the remaining cheese on the top so it melts.

When cooked, serve as is or preferred toppings (sugar free ketchup, salsa, etc.).

This will have around 290/300 calories, 2g of fat, 22g of carbs, 5g of fiber and 44g of protein.

Egg White Avo Toast & Egg Avo Toast

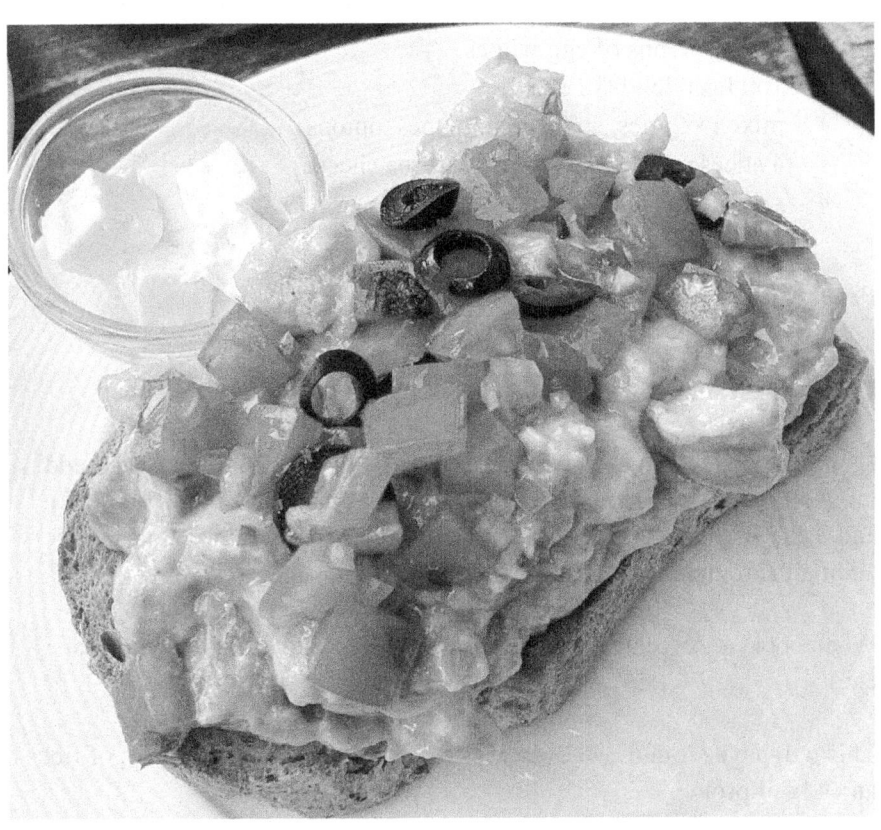

Egg White Avo Toast

You think avocado makes you fat? Not really. It is a really great source of healthy fats, like the ones you really need for your body.

Difficulty: ✪

Ingredients:

- 2 slices of bread.
- 60g of avocado
- 90g of sliced tomato
- 40g of chopped onion and tomato
- 1 cup or 240g of egg whites
- 3 minced cloves of garlic
- 1tsp paprika
- 1tsp of lemon juice.

Preparation:

Make some guac out of that avocado and add the seasonings, tomato, garlic etc. and mix, then toast the bread.
Heat a pan over medium-high heat, spray with cooking spray and cook egg whites.
Serve as follows: add the guac Avo paste on top of toasty bread and then cooked egg white on top either as a 2 open piece toas or as a big tall sando.

430 cal, 12g of fat, 54g of carbs, 14g of fiber and 35g of protein

For the Egg Avo Toast

Same ingredients as the Egg white Avo toast, just change the 1 cup of egg whites for 3/4 cup of egg whites and 2 whole eggs.

Calories are 550, 21g fat, 50g carbs, 10g fiber, 44g protein

Egg White Bites

This Vegetarian and Gluten Free should be ready in 20 mins or so.

Difficulty: ✪

Ingredients:

- 480g or 2 cups of egg whites
- 100g of spinach
- 100g of tomatoes diced.
- 4 slices of fat free cheese or 70g of shredded fat free cheese

Preparation:

1 - Preheat oven for 400F/204C.
2 - In a bowl, whisk egg whites, cheese, salt, and pepper to taste.
3 - Spray nonstick muffin pan with spray.
4 - Stuff spinach leaves into each mold, add tomatoes and carefully fill with egg white mix.
5 - Bake for 10 mins or until cooked and that's it!

410 calories, 1g of fat, 23g of carbs, 4g of fiber and 72g of protein

Protein Muffins (Blueberry)

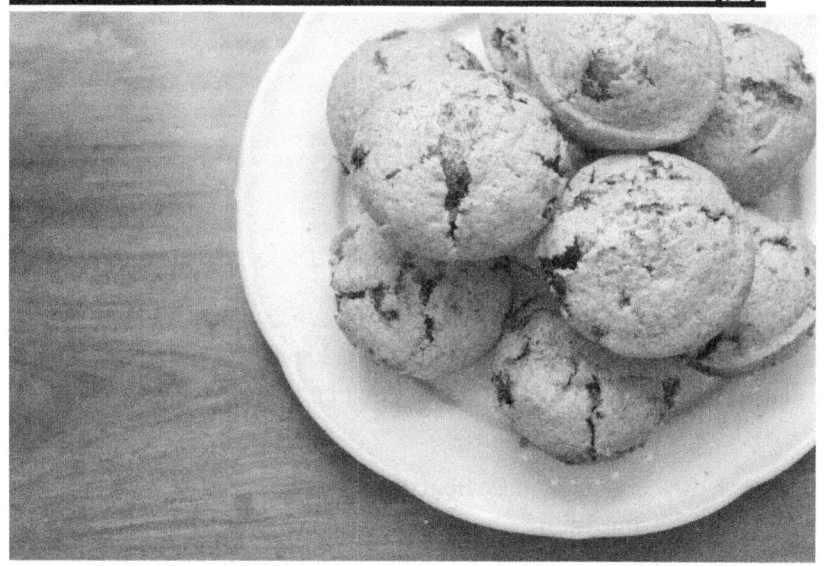

Yeah buddy, you'll be having muffins for breakfast. These ones are healthy!

Difficulty: ✪

Ingredients:

- 1 cup or 250g of unsweetened apple sauce
- 180g or 3/4 cup of 0% fat free Greek yogurt.
- 60g or 1/4 cup of egg whites.
- 2 scoops of preferred protein powder
- 2 cups or 240g of oat flour
- 270g fresh blueberries
- 1 tsp or 5g of vanilla extract
- 6 packets of sweetener
- 6g or 1 1/2 of baking powder
- 4g or 1/2 tsp of baking soda

Preparation

Preheat oven to 325F or 163C and while that is happening, combine all wet ingredients until perfectly mixed on one bowl and the dry ones on another bowl as well.

Combine both dry and wet ingredients together until it is smooth. Add blueberries. Spray a muffin tray with cooking spray and pour this batter to the muffin tray and leave around half an inch or close to 1cm to room for the muffins to rise.

Bake this mixture for 15 to 20 mins or until they look nicey-nice from the screen of the oven. Let them cool and serve!

This batch has 1620 calories, 23g of fat, 240g of carbs, 33g of fiber and 119g of protein. Each muffin will have around 160 cal, 2g of fat, 24g of carbs, 3g of fiber and 12g of protein.

Lunch

Chili Chicken Rice Bowls:

This recipe is for 5 servings, so consider making this for your lunch over a work week. That's what I do.

Difficulty: ✪✪✪

Ingredients:

- 3 cups (450 g) cooked rice
- 2 lbs. (908 g) boneless skinless chicken thighs
- ⅔ cup (150 g) plain nonfat Greek yogurt
- 1 tbsp (8 g) chili powder
- 1 tbsp (8 g) onion powder
- 1 tbsp (8 g) garlic powder
- 1 tsp (6 g) salt
- 1 tbsp (15 g) lemon juice
- 2 medium (300 g) bell peppers any color.
- 1 small (125 g) onion
- 12 oz (340 g) shredded cabbage.
- 1 (20 g) chili pepper optional
- 1 tsp (3 g) onion powder
- 1 tsp (3 g) chili powder
- 2 tbsp (30 g) oil
- 1 tbsp (15 g) minced garlic.
- 1 tbsp (15 g) lemon juice
- 8 oz (227 g) tomato sauce

Preparation:

First, Prep the Chicken:

- Into a large bowl, add the Greek yogurt, 1 tbsp each of onion powder, garlic powder, chili powder and lemon juice, as well as 1 tsp of salt. Mix to combine.
- Add in the chicken thighs and coat all the cracks and crevices of the chicken with the yogurt marinade.
- Cook in an air fryer on 400F for 12 mins or until cooked.
- Remove and let rest and then cut into dices.

Second, Prep the Rice:

- Cook enough rice to yield 3 cups (450g) of cooked rice. 1 cup of dry rice will make between 2-3 cups of rice depending on what kind you use.

Third, Prep the Vegetables:

- Wash and cut all your vegetables to prepare for cooking. Cut the peppers and the onion into a medium dice.
- Mince some garlic until you have 1 tbsp worth.
- For the cabbage I use the shredded stuff in the bag. If you buy a head of cabbage, shred it into thin slices.
- For the chili, you can use a jalapeño, serrano, or a red chili if you decide to use one. It is not necessary for this recipe but if you would like a bit more heat, cut one into a small dice and add it to the vegetables.
- In a large skillet over medium heat, add about 1 tbsp of oil. Once the oil is hot, add in the onion powder and chili powder and allow the spices to bloom for about 30 seconds.
- Add in the remaining 1 tbsp of oil if needed and dump in your onions and peppers. Season lightly with salt and mix the spices into the vegetables.
- Cook the vegetables for about 3-5 minutes and then add in the shredded cabbage and garlic. Mix to combine and cook for about 1-2 minutes.
- Add in the tomato sauce and stir into the vegetables. Allow this to cook for 3-5 minutes and cook out the raw tomato flavor.
- Add in 3 cups (450g) of cooked rice, all the diced chicken, 1 tbsp of lemon juice, and salt and pepper to taste.

This will make 5 servings, and each should have 470 calories, 42g of carbs, 42g of protein and 11g of fat.

QUESADILLA

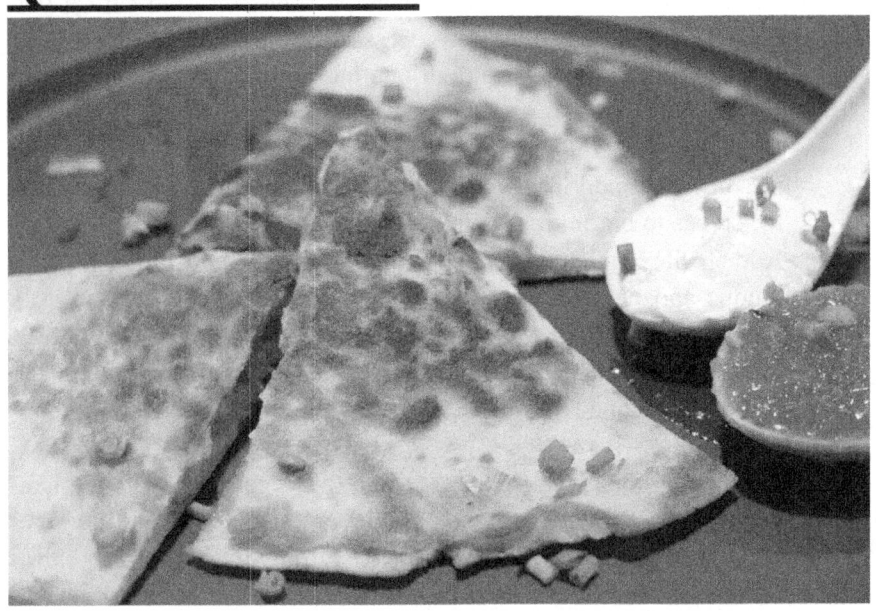

Who doesn't like a quesadilla? This is a healthier version of it, so check it out!

Difficulty: ✪

Ingredients:

- 60g of any type of meat preferred (make sure it's lean)
- 2 low carb high fiber tortilla
- 2 slices of fat free cheese
- veggies to assist (peppers/onions/jalapeños/mushrooms)
- Salsa and sour cream (fat free) for toppings

Preparation:

- Prepare meat as preferred (I'd grill it) with salt pepper or seasonings you prefer to taste and have it ready (you can refrigerate).
- You can do this if you have a big enough pan on the stove, if not, preheat the oven to 375GF, add foil, add spray, place one tortilla, spread all veggies, cheese and meat even on top of it and add other tortilla on top
- Bake or cook for 5 to 10 mins or until desired doneness.
- Slice like a quesadilla and that's all folks.

This should be around 350 cal, 8g of fat, 60 of carbs, 35 of fiber and 30 of protein.

TACO PASTA

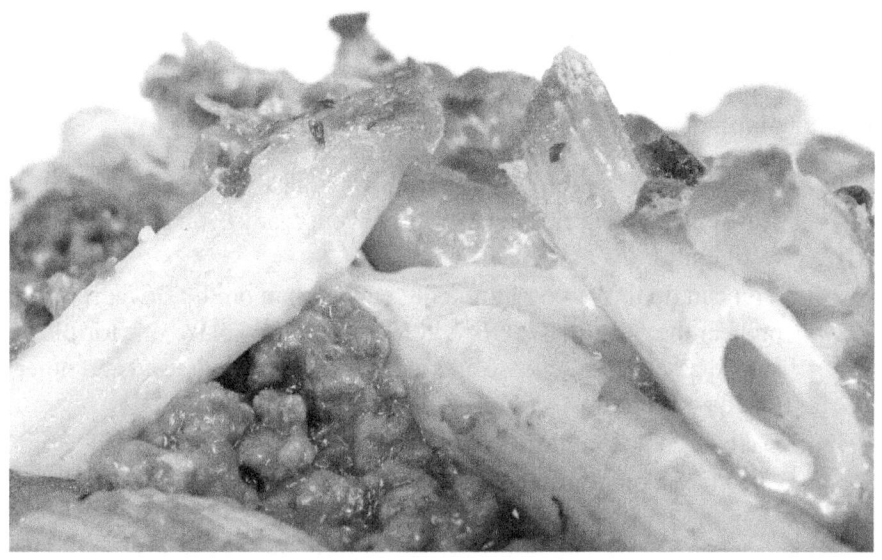

That name makes no sense I know but hear me out. A pasta dish that tastes like taco bell? This is it. This is for 5 servings as well.

Difficulty: ✪✪✪

Ingredients:

- 2 pounds lean ground turkey
- 3tsp garlic salt
- 3tsp cumin
- 3tsp onion powder
- 3tsp paprika
- 2tsp cayenne pepper
- 2tsp coriander
- 2tbsp cornstarch
- 120ml water
- salt and pepper to taste.
- 1 onion diced.
- 1 pound of elbows or preferred pasta.

Preparation:

First, Prep the Meat:

In a medium bowl, combine the beef, garlic salt, cumin, onion powder, paprika, cayenne, and coriander. Cover and refrigerate for 30 minutes. Spray Cooking spray on a large skillet over medium-high.

Add the diced onion and cook until softened and translucent. Add the seasoned and marinated meat now and cook, breaking up the pieces with, until browned, 5 to 7 minutes.

Mix the cornstarch with ½ cup|120 ml water and add to the beef; bring to a boil. Cook, uncovered and stirring occasionally, until thick, about 4 minutes. Season with salt and pepper and keep warm.

Second, Prep Pasta

Cook pasta as per instructions, remove from heat when done and drain.

Add pasta to meat and mix. You now have a pasta turkey that taste like seasoned taco meat for the week.

This should do 5 servings. Each should be 420 cal, 41g protein, 14g of fat, 2g of fiber, and 35g of carbs

Chipotle Chicken & Rice

Spicy stuff? You got it. This is also for 5 servings.

Difficulty: ✪✪✪

Ingredients

- 2 lbs (908 g) boneless skinless chicken thighs
- 1½ tbsp (23 g) olive oil
- 1 medium (150 g) red bell pepper
- 1 medium (150 g) green bell pepper
- 1 medium (200 g) onion
- 3½ cups (525 g) cooked rice
- 1 tbsp (15 g) lime juice
- 4 tbsp (60 g) chipotle peppers in adobo sauce
- 1 tsp (3 g) garlic powder
- salt and pepper to taste.

Preparation:

First, Prep the Rice:

- Cook enough rice to yield 3½ cups of cooked rice. 1 cup of dry rice will yield between 2-3 cups of cooked rice.

Second, Prep the Chicken:

- I prefer to cook this in the air fryer. If you don't have one you can use the bake and broil method in the oven. Preheat your air fryer to 400°F or your oven to 425°F.
- Cut the chipotle peppers into a mince with some of the adobo sauce until you have about ¼ cup worth.
- Season the chicken with salt and pepper and add about 2 tbsp of the chipotle peppers and adobo sauce. Toss the chicken to coat with the sauce.
- Place the chicken into your air fryer basket and air fry for 8-12 minutes.

Third, Prep Veggies:

- Wash and cut your peppers into a large dice.
- Cut the onion into slices.
- In a large skillet, heat some oil over medium high heat.
- Add the onions and cook for 4-5 minutes until they have begun to caramelize.
- Add more oil if needed and add in the peppers.
- Season with salt to help bring out some of the moisture.
- Cook for 3-4 minutes and remove from the pan.

Finally,

- Cut the chicken into a medium dice.
- Into a large skillet, add the chicken and allow it to develop a bit more color on all sides.
- Add in the peppers and onions, the cooked rice, and the remaining chipotle peppers.
- Toss to coat evenly.
- Add the garlic powder and lime juice.
- Stir to incorporate and season with salt and pepper to taste.

This will make 5 servings. Each with 500 calories, 39g of carbs, 47g of Protein and 18g of fat.

Vegan Meatball Sub

This is an easy sub that you can make right away. High protein and ready to eat immediately.

Difficulty: ✪

Ingredients:

- 2 slices of protein bread (140 calories per slice)
- 4 veggie meatballs (120 cal)
- veggies (onion, lettuce, tomato)
- mustard, sugar free ketchup

Preparation:

Heat up meatballs in microwave according to directions, toast bread slices and build accordingly. Top with preferred condiments or vegies. See how easy it is?

This easy to make dish should be around 430 calories, 15g of fat, 43g of carbs, 8g fiber, 45g protein. If you use regular bread is 310 cal and half the protein.

Deconstructed Cheeseburger

If someone tells you a cheeseburger isn't healthy. Eat this one and prove them wrong.

Difficulty: ✪✪✪

Ingredients

- 3 medium (750 g) russet potatoes
- 2 lbs. (908 g) ground beef (Lean)
- 1 bunch (125 g) kale
- 1 small (125 g) red onion
- 2 spears (50 g) dill pickles
- 1 tbsp (15 g) oil
- 1 tbsp (8 g) garlic powder
- salt and pepper to taste.
- ½ cup (50 g) shredded cheddar cheese

Preparation:

First, Prep the Potatoes:

- Preheat your oven to 425°F. Place your sheet pans inside while it preheats.
- Wash and cut your potatoes into a large dice.
- Add the potatoes to a large bowl with 1 tbsp of oil and salt and pepper to taste.
- Spray the sheet pan lightly with oil and spread the potatoes out evenly.
- Roast for 10-12 minutes then flip the potatoes to the other side and continue cooking for an additional 8-10 minutes or until they have browned to your liking.

Second, Prep the Cheeseburger:

- Cut your onion into thin slices from root to shoot.
- Wash and remove the kale leaves from the stems. Roughly chop the kale into smaller pieces.
- Massage the chopped kale for a few minutes by squeezing it in your hands.
- Cut the pickle spears into a small dice.
- In a large skillet, heat 1 tbsp of oil over medium high heat and add in your beef to brown. Spread it out in the bottom of the skillet and allow it to develop color before you break it up.
- When it is ready to turn, flip it over to the other side and now you can start to break it up.
- When the beef is about 90% of the way finished, move it to the perimeter of your pan and allow the fat to pool in the center.
- Add the onions to the middle and sprinkle a bit of salt over the top to encourage them to cook faster.
- After a minute or two and the onions have had a chance on the heat, dump the kale into the skillet and season with 1 tbsp of garlic powder.
- Mix the contents of the skillet together and allow the kale and onions to continue to cook.
- When the potatoes have finished, add them to skillet and mix. Taste test and season with salt and pepper to taste.

Divide and serve with some no sugar added ketchup

Makes 5 servings - Each serving is around 580 Cal, 41g Carbs, 43g Protein and 28g fat

Open Face Chicken Sando x2

I couldn't talk about the cheeseburger without mentioning the Chicken Sandwich, right? Here you go for a healthier spin on this one.

Difficulty: ✪✪

Ingredients:

- 2 slices of bread (80 cals per slice)
- 160g chicken breast or thigh/cooked.
- Preferred spices (ms dash, garlic powder, paprika, salt and pepper, etc)
- Canned gravy (60 cals per 3/4 cup)

Preparation:

Heat a griddle over med heat and add chicken to cook on both sides with your spices to taste until cooked through.

Heat up gravy. Place the chicken breasts over the 2 slices of bread and top with gravy.

This should be around 505 cal, 13g fat, 39g carbs, 2g fiber 50g protein.

Snacks & Appetizers

Popcorn

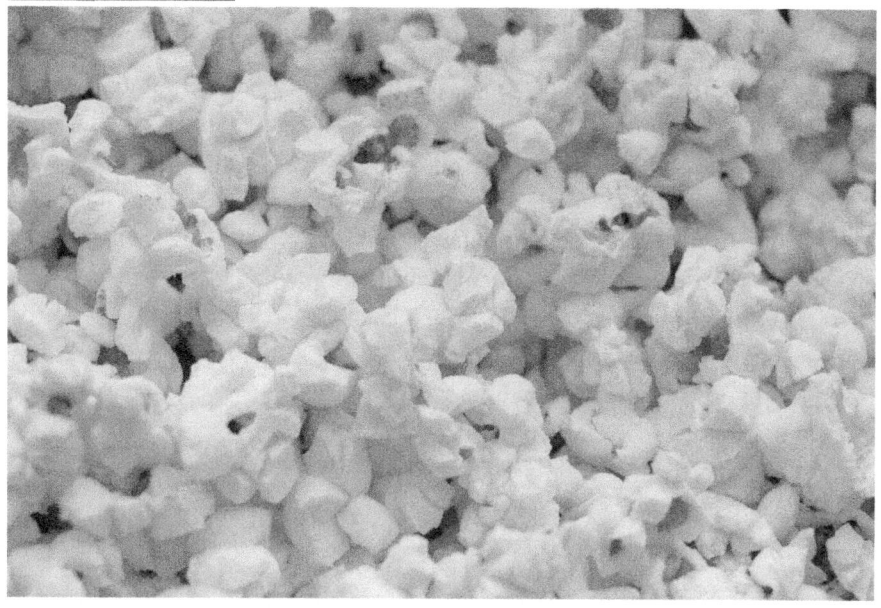

Ingredients and Preparation:

Buy raw popcorn, prepare it as you prefer (I use a microwave bowl), and add seasonings to it! this will fill you up more than any bag of chips with less than a third of the calories!

PeaNOT Butter cupcakes

Cupcakes healthy? Whaaat?

Difficulty: ✪

Ingredients:

- 60g of powdered peanut butter
- 2 scoops of preferred chocolate protein powder
- 375g of chickpeas (rinsed from a can)
- 20g sugar free chocolate chips
- 60g or 1/4 cup of egg whites.
- 175g of nonfat Greek yogurt
- 15g or 1tbsp of vanilla extract
- 1/4 tsp of salt
- 2 packets of sweeteners
- 60ml or syrup
- 1/2 tsp of baking powder

Preparation:

- Preheat oven to 350F. blend all ingredients except chips until smooth, then add chips into mix.
- Add mixture to cupcake or baking pan and bake for 15 mins or so that's it.

One serving is 165 calories, 4g of fat, 18g of carbs, 4g of fiber and 16g of protein. Whole batch should be 8 times that

RICE CAKES!

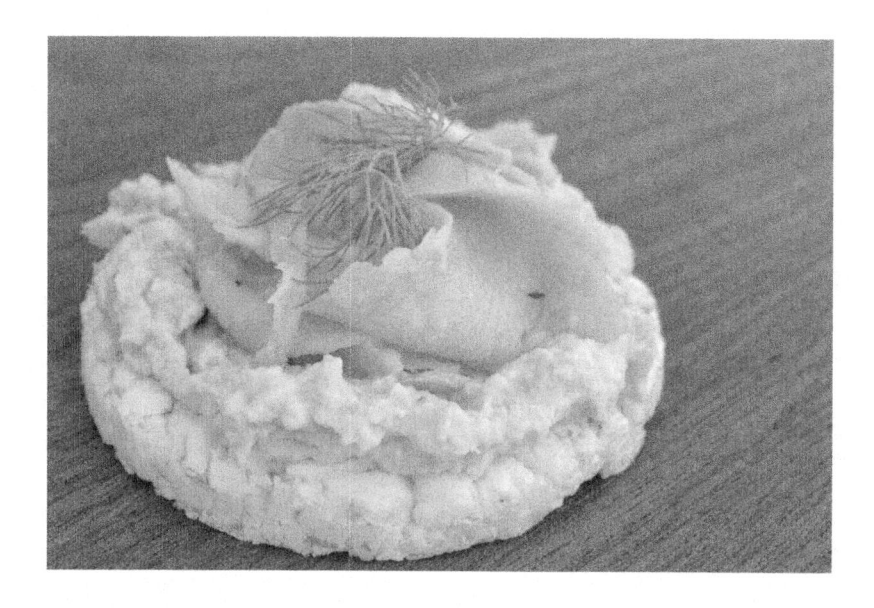

Ingredients and Preparation:

Buy rice cakes and add some healthy fats and proteins to make it a snack, you can add avocado, salmon or even deli meat and you're good to go!

Protein Fruit Ice Cream

Now Ice cream? Hell yeah brother. Ice cream can be made healthy with the right ingredients. Check this out:

Difficulty: ✪

Ingredients:

- 1 scoop of protein powder of choice
- 45g of blueberries
- 1g or 1/4tsb of guar gum
- 90ml or unsweet almond milk
- Ice

Preparation:

Add all ingredients to a blender, blend 1 min on med speed until smooth, make sure to stop and scrape sides until everything is incorporated. Pulsing helps and always add more ice or milk to achieve a consistency you prefer. I recommend eating this right away.

A serving should be around 185 Cal, 3g of fat, 14g of carbs, 4g of fiber and 26g of protein

Cauliflower mash

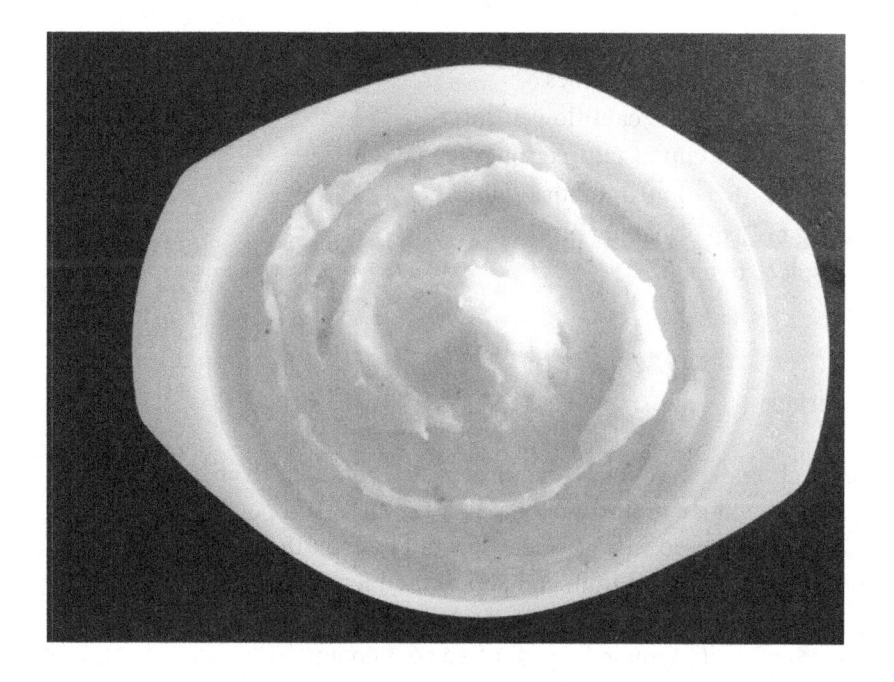

This will taste even better than regular mashed potatoes.

Difficulty: ✪✪✪

Ingredients:

- 900g or 2lbs of potatoes
- 900g or 2lbs of cauliflower florets
- 530g or 1 cup of fat free sour cream.
- 9g or 3tsp of guar/xanthan gum
- 8g or 2tsp of baking powder
- spices to taste

Preparation

Boil enough water (around 4 liters) of water with salt over high heat and when it boils, reduce to medium heat to a simmer. Add potatoes in pot until cooked, drain and add to a blender. Separately cook the cauliflower florets in a boiling pot of water, train and add to the blender. Add baking powder, half of the fat free sour cream and guar gum to blender and pulse until smooth. Serve with remainder of fat free sour cream.

Per serving you should have 150 calories, no fat, 34g of carbs, 8g of fiber and 5g of protein.

Egg white fries

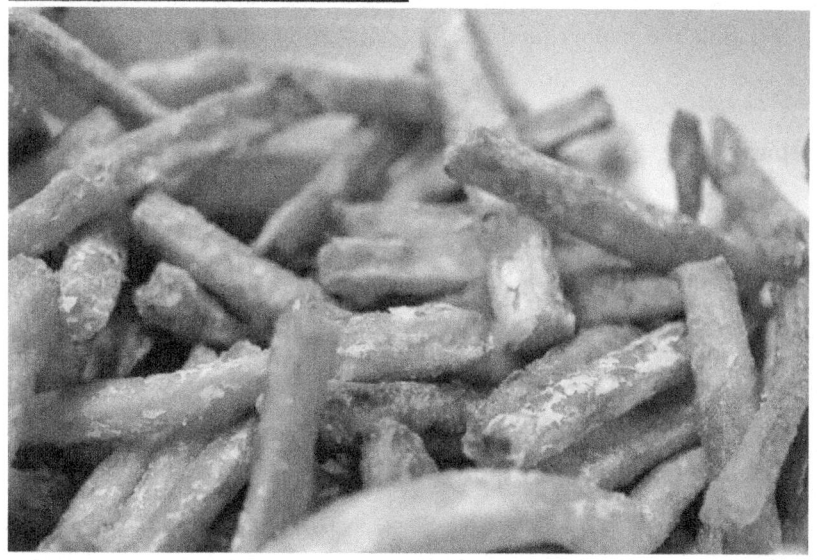

I hope you see now that there are no limits to this game. Now we have fries!

Difficulty: ✪

Ingredients:

- 175g of white or russet potatoes
- 115g of sweet potato
- 120g or 1/2cup of egg whites
- Salt and pepper (and add any other spices you prefer)

Preparation:

- Preheat oven to 400F/204C and cut the potatoes lengthwise into fried shapes.
- Place in a bowl and add egg white over the potatoes and sprinkle with seasonings.
- Place foil or parchment paper on a baking sheet, spray with cooking spray and place the fries on top.
- Bake for 20 mins, remove, and then move them around on the tray and cook again for 10 more mins. Remove again, let cool and enjoy!

Servings should be around 330 calories, 1g of fat, 60g of carbs, 8g of fiber and 20g of protein.

Homemade Chicken Nuggets

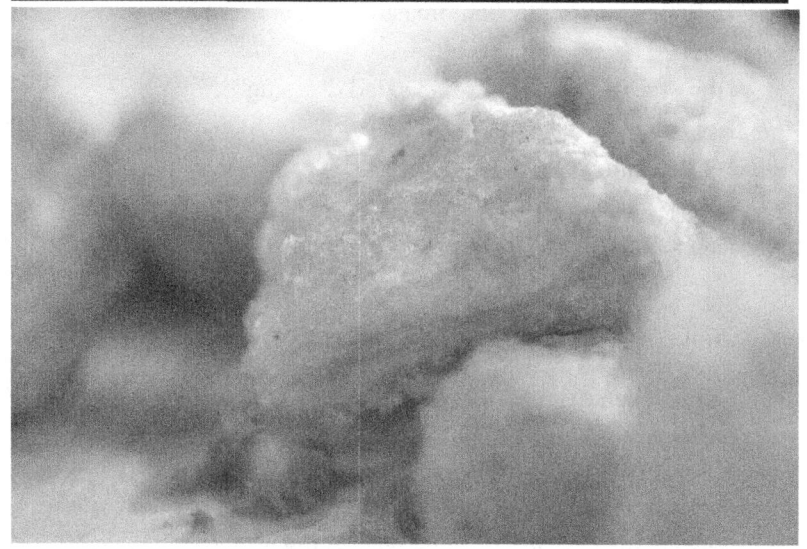

Not as good as the real thing, but close and waaay healthier.

Difficulty: ✪

Ingredients:

- 454g or 16oz of chicken breast or thighs
- 60g or 1/4 cup of egg whites.
- 1tbsp fat free or light Italian salad dressing
- 1 tsp paprika
- 1/4 tsp cumin
- 1/2 tsp garlic powder
- 1tsp salt

Preparation:

- Cut chicken to small pieces and put in a bowl, pour salad dressing, and mix and then save for a couple of hours.
- Pour egg whites into another bowl then add the chicken pieces to the egg whites and add the spices.
- Place in air frier for 10 mins over at the air fryer for like 10 mins and that's it

Servings should be around 500 Cal, 12g of fat, 5g of carbs, 1g of fiber and 92g of protein.

DINNERS

Swed(ish) Meatballs

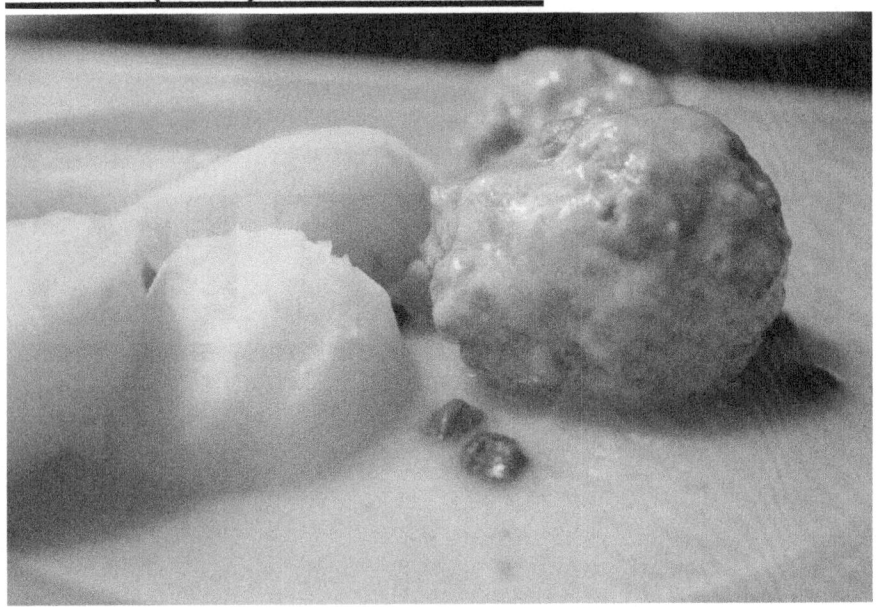

Now let's pretend we go to Ikea and these are from there. Imagine this being the healthier version of those.

Difficulty: ✪✪

Ingredients:

- 900g or 32oz of lean ground turkey or beef
- 160g of panko breadcrumbs
- 960ml beef broth
- 30g or 4 tbsp of corn starch
- 60ml or 4 tbsp of water
- Salt, black pepper, and garlic powder to taste. You can add cinnamon, nutmeg, onion powder.
- 1/2 tsp clove

Preparation:

- In a large bowl, add meat, breadcrumbs, spices and mix thoroughly to make sure the meat gets all spices.
- Portion out meatball mix (around 20 meatballs) and place them on a baking sheet tray coated with spray.
- Preheat oven to 400F/204C and bake the meatballs in the oven for over 20 mins or cooked internally to 165F, remove, and let them rest.
- In a skillet, add beef broth over high heat – on another bowl, mix corn starch and water to make a slurry.
- When beef stock is boiling, add slurry and whisk until it thickens to your desire way and then add the meatballs.

That's it, serve as is and add parsley for garnish if you want. Mix with some of the appetizers mentioned before and you're in for a treat.

Total batch is 2150 calories, 78g of fat, 168g of carbs, 5g of fiber and 194 of protein. Divide by the number of meatballs and you'll have your individual numbers.

Citrusy Tilapia and Shrimp

I thought a bit of fish needed to be incorporated into this thing. So, let's check this one out:

Difficulty: ✪

Ingredients:

- 850g or 30oz of tilapia filet
- 425g of peeled shrimp
- 550g zucchini in strips
- 550g green shredded cabbage
- 300g of diced tomatoes
- 550g of yellow squash in strips
- 300g of carrots in trips
- 5 minced garlic cloves
- 50g yellow onion minced.
- zest and juice of 5 lemons
- salt pepper to taste.
- 5tbsp of water

Preparation:

- Heat a skillet over high heat, spray cooking spray, add all veggies and toss and cook with salt and pepper.
- Sautee until ALMOST cooked.
- Preheat oven to 400F or 204C, spray baking sheet with parchment paper with cooking spray and lay tilapia filets there and pour all lemon juice over all of them.
- Transfer shrimp and sauteed veggies on top of these filets and cook for 10 mins or so or until you notice tilapia is fully cooked.
- Remove from oven and serve.

Serving should be 380 calories, 5g of fat, 30g of carbs, 8g of fiber and 57g of protein.

Baked salmon & Long Greens

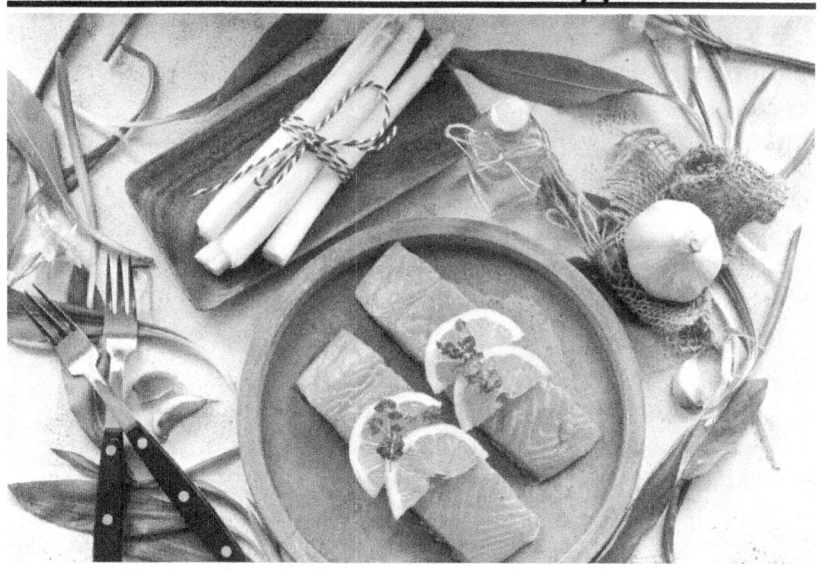

This will be the fancy dinner for your anniversary or something, but in a healthier way.

Difficulty: ✪

Ingredients:

- 1000g or 35oz of salmon
- 1000g of asparagus
- 500g of diced yellow onion.
- 2 cloves of minced garlic
- 1 lemon
- salt, pepper garlic powder

Preparation:

- Preheat oven to 450F/232C and separately in a bowl add the asparagus, garlic, onions, and lemon zest with salt to taste and black pepper.
- Spray with cooking spray and toss well.
- Season salmon with salt, pepper, and garlic powder to taste and place on a baking sheet (add lemon slices on top of salmon) also add the asparagus on that sheet too.
- Bake all this for 12 mins or until everything is cooked through and serve!

Serving should be 425 calories, 20g of fat, 16 of carbs, 4 of fiber and 40 of protein. The whole batch should be like 5 or 6 times that.

PIZZA A LA PROTEINA

Cheeseburgers, Chicken Sandwiches, Fries and now Pizza. Yeah, you can make anything using healthier stuff!

Difficulty: ✪

Ingredients:

- P28 Hight protein flat bread or Joseph's Lavash Bread
- 50g of lean ground meat
- slices of cheese or fat free mozzarella
- Peppers, onions, mushrooms, spinach.
- Sugar Free Ketchup or preferred marinara or pizza sauce.

Preparation

- First, toast the flat bread for 3 mins in oven for 300F.
- Second, take out of oven and add half a cup or less of pizza sauce to coat it.
- Then add cheese slices or shredded, add ground meat and toppings back to oven to 4 or 5 mins and that's it!

You do the math for the servings on this one as practice from what we have learned on this book.

Epilogue:

Hope you enjoyed it. Again, I tried to make it easy. Not too many recipes, all easy to do, in a short book, all as a lazy person would do. So go ahead and start making these.

The thing with cookbooks and recipes and stuff like that is that they fail. If you enjoyed any of these, start changing one of your meals to one of these and you FOR SURE will lose weight. Hope these recipes take you on an insightful introspection where you will be able to get to know yourself better. Just make it a lifestyle.

If you liked it and found it helpful, recommend it to a friend! I was able to just shed pounds and improve my health by eating better and just walking. The more you weight, the more weight you will lose and that's a fact. Or science or something. If you liked this book, remember to check my site (www.miguelrecs.com) and donate so I can buy Leo and Layla more toys.

Cheers,

Miguel L.

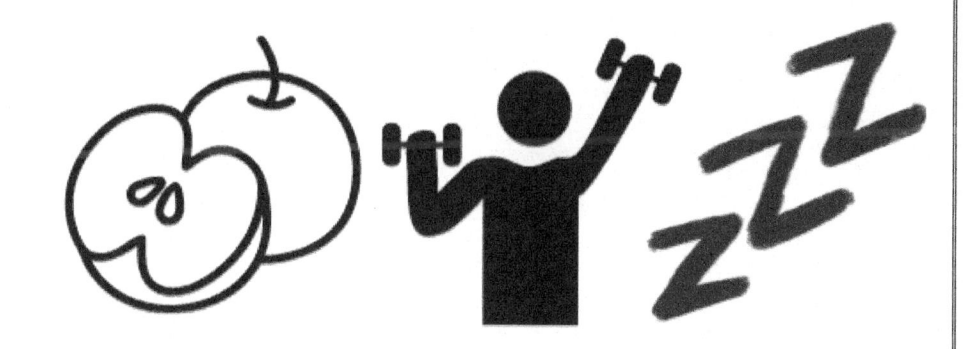

Made in United States
Orlando, FL
04 October 2025